coping with serious illness

Catherine Thornton

VERITAS

First published 2007 by
Veritas Publications
7/8 Lower Abbey Street
Dublin 1
Ireland

Email publications@veritas.ie
Website www.veritas.ie

ISBN 978 1 84730 051 5

'Beannacht' by John O'Donohue taken from *Anam Cara*,
courtesy of Bantam Books, 1997.

'Everything is going to be alright' by Derek Mahon taken
from *Selected Poems*, new ed., courtesy of Penguin, 2001.

A catalogue record for this book is available from the
British Library.

Printed in the Republic of Ireland by Betaprint Ltd, Dublin

Veritas books are printed on paper made from the wood
pulp of managed forests. For every tree felled, at least one
tree is planted, thereby renewing natural resources.

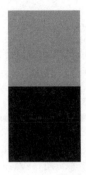

Contents

Dedication

I believe that we draw great comfort from each other and it is others who lift us up and carry us on when we cannot do so ourselves.

I would like to thank all those who have carried me over the years – you know who you are and I would not be here without you.

The poem 'Beannacht' by John O'Donohue expresses better than I could what I wish for you.

> On the day when
> the weight deadens
> on your shoulders
> and you stumble,
> may the clay dance
> to balance you.

And when your eyes
freeze behind
the grey window
and the ghost of loss
gets in to you,
may a flock of colours,
indigo, red, green,
and azure blue
come to awaken in you
a meadow of delight.

When the canvas frays
in the currach of thought
and a stain of ocean
blackens beneath you,
may there come across the
waters
a path of yellow moonlight
to bring you safely home.

May the nourishment of the
earth be yours,
may the clarity of light be yours,
may the fluency of the ocean be
yours,
may the protection of the
ancestors be yours.

coping with serious illness

And so may a slow
wind work these words
of love around you,
an invisible cloak
to mind your life.

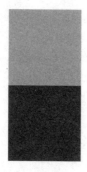

Introduction

Seven years ago I was diagnosed with breast cancer.

I was forty-five years old, had been married for twenty years and had three sons. I was busy and didn't have time for such things in my life. But I had to make time. Things changed for me; some changes were temporary, some permanent.

My illness came on suddenly and required a drastic and fairly speedy reaction. It involved surgery, invasive medicines and a change to my body shape that attacked the very basis of how I saw myself as a woman. There was all the physical and emotional turmoil that comes with any diagnosis of a serious illness; there was also the difficulty of having to deal with how others saw me. I became part of the medical system, which was a new and strange experience

My family were also affected. My husband and sons definitely, but also my mother and sister. My sister had been similarly diagnosed three years previously and now had to deal with this all over again. My mother had to look at another daughter going down this road.

It is now seven years on from that November day when I first heard the word 'cancer' related to me. I lived through the operation and the treatments and am back leading my normal day-to-day life. I still have to live with my body as it is now and learn to love it. I also have to return regularly to the various clinics to keep an eye on the cancer, to make sure it isn't coming back.

Most days I count my blessings and thank God I am still here and healthy, relatively speaking, but to be honest there are days when I resent that I had this illness and that I have to live within the boundaries it has set for me. However, my getting ill has been part of my life experience, part of what I am today, and I value it for that.

In illness we cry, but we also, hopefully, find laughter, friendship and spiritual comfort. Many people helped me on my journey, got me to where I am today and made the bad days a little better. This book is a record of that journey, of my hopes and my fears, of the different lessons I learned on the way. I had cancer but I think what I am saying will apply to any serious life-changing illness. I don't have all the answers but I would like to share my experiences in the hope that they can be of help to others. I have always found it helpful to read about how others have dealt with difficulties they encounter in their lives and what helped them along the way. I feel that we can all learn from each other and hearing people talk about their experiences makes us realise that we are not alone.

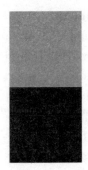

chapter 1

Dealing with the Diagnosis

Nobody expects serious illness to happen to them. When it does we all react in different ways. Some look it straight in the eye and say 'Bring it on!'; others bury their head in the sand, hoping that if they hide for long enough it will disappear.

Serious illness can come when we are young or in middle or old age. It decides the time – we don't. It nearly always begins unexpectedly but then inevitably has to be faced. The one thing we do know is that it isn't like a cold, the flu or even a hospital stay for a serious operation.

For me what defines it is the uncertainty about when it will end – a future that is usually neither immediately apparent nor predictable. We won't be sick for just a few weeks and then go into recovery. We won't get back to normal life. Our normal life is going to be redefined: from now on it will most likely include visiting the hospital regularly, taking medicines and possibly losing our independence.

There are so many serious illnesses that it would be impossible for me to talk about all the changes that they bring to our lives. There are also so many individual reactions that it would also be impossible and even impertinent of me to suggest what would be an appropriate reaction to a diagnosis. The only thing we can say for sure is that the illness is going to change our lives whether in a greater or smaller measure. It is also going to change the lives of those around us who love us and want to care for and help us. The other thing it changes is the way some people look at us.

When I got a diagnosis of a serious illness I was a storm of emotions. I was frightened, angry and suddenly unsure of my future. I was no longer in control. Now I know that none of us are totally in charge of our own destiny, yet we feel that we make the decisions to some extent. Serious illness takes us into a new area. Now decisions very important to our life will be made with the advice of strangers, granted very experienced and learned strangers, but nevertheless people we don't know.

We are starting out on a journey that we didn't plan and didn't ask to go on. We don't know our ultimate destination but we need to know the map and study it in order to have some sense of where we are being brought and what we ourselves can do to help reach the desired destination.

At a class I was attending a few weeks after my diagnosis, a woman gave us all little cards with 'thought-provoking' sayings on them. I took one with indifference but when I turned it over it read 'the future has a way of arriving unannounced'. Over the coming weeks trying to come to terms with my future I often thought about these few simple words and what they meant.

I knew from the first time that a doctor said out loud what I knew in my heart, a future that I hadn't planned for had arrived. From that day plans I had would be put on hold for an indeterminate length of time. I walked from that hospital room in a daze, feeling that I had stepped over some invisible line from one part of the population to another. I was now officially a sick person, someone for whom a team would meet to discuss a plan of action. I felt helpless and lost.

Up to that moment I had defined myself in different ways depending on my mood: I was a wife, mother, daughter, sister, friend and busy member of the community within which I lived. I was a woman moving towards middle age trying to redefine myself in those terms, thinking of the time when my family would be reared, thinking of the future. I was contemplating a possible return to work, to study and new vistas ahead.

Now there was a new definition: a woman who was sick; a woman who could die. After the shock came the anger. I shouted the universal question of the ill: 'Why me? What have I done to deserve this?' I felt that God, who, up to now, had been fairly good to me, had let me down. I had people dependent on me, I had a life I was enjoying. There was no room for illness in this!

Many days of endless cycles of thought led me to another question: 'Why not me?' Every day people fall ill, receive an unwanted diagnosis that changes their lives; why should I be special and be given an amnesty on suffering?

The next step was deciding what to do. There were two paths open: I could sit down and fearfully wait for the illness to do its worst, to leave the arena before the fight began, or I could to decide to do battle with all the tools available. I decided on the latter. My life was worth fighting for and I would use all the expertise available, all the help on offer – spiritual, emotional and physical – to try to beat the illness. I might not be the same person or have the ability to do all the things I used to do, but I would try to be the best I could. The diagnosis would be the beginning of a journey not the end.

> The more serious the illness, the more important it is for you to fight back, mobilising all your resources, emotional, intellectual, physical.
>
> (Norman Cousins)

> I learned that courage was not the absence of fear, but the triumph over it. The brave man is not he who does not feel

afraid, but he who conquers that fear.

(Nelson Mandela)

MAIN POINTS

Everyone's reaction to an initial diagnosis is different – there is no right or wrong way to react.

We have no control over what the future brings but we can decide how to deal with it.

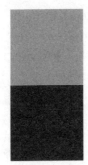

chapter 2

Interacting with the Medical System

Every time I have an appointment with a health professional for a check up I come home from it feeling exhausted. I worry that all will go okay and hope that I won't hear something unwelcome. I also find it a stressful experience. Before I go I make notes for myself of any questions I want to ask. I know that if I don't have them written down I will forget them. I also take a list of my appointments with other doctors and what tests I have had and when they were done.

When I have this information with me it means that at least I feel I will be able to answer the questions that are inevitably put to me. Perhaps the doctors should know the details, but they arrive clutching my hospital folder, which by this time is several inches thick with many loose pieces of paper protruding untidily. A lot of valuable time can be lost waiting for them to leaf through this for the relevant information for the day's consultation. Maybe the hospital should have a more information-age system available, but it doesn't, so some time ago I decided that I would benefit by coming prepared to my appointments. This is just one of the ways that helps me to feel more in control of the situation.

When I was finally diagnosed with cancer seven years ago, I had already dealt with many doctors and other health professionals during that short journey from first worry to diagnosis. This was to be the start of a long relationship with a series of people who were to play a big part in how my future would work out. These people are strangers yet I would have to put huge trust in them. I would have to listen to the advice they were giving me and decide how to act on it.

When you are ill you don't want to have to learn something new, yet this is what I needed to do in order to feel that I was still in charge of my life. Health professionals use a lot of words that are very familiar to them yet are totally unfamiliar to the rest of us. They don't do this to confuse us, sometimes they don't even realise that they have lost us in the conversation, but if we don't speak up we will end up becoming more distanced from an understanding of what is happening. I felt a need during the intense part of my illness, and still do, to know what was happening and why. So much of our lives goes out of our control when we are ill that it is good to exercise some control when we can.

The doctors are there to help us, to make us feel better, and in nearly all cases they are happy to answer our questions. There is no shame in admitting that we don't understand what they are saying and asking them to explain it again. At these times we can be feeling scared, confused and tired, so it is good to bring somebody else with us when we see the doctor. Two sets of ears are always better and they may hear something that we have missed.

When a doctor asks us how we are feeling today, it is not like the casual inquiry from someone we meet at the shops. Unlike that person, the doctor does actually want to know how we are. If we say, 'Fine thanks, doctor', how are they supposed to know that the tablets we are on are making us miserable or that we have that ache we are worried about? Nothing is too silly to ask about and the relief you can get from a reassuring answer or a discussion about medication is incredible.

I felt more in control of my illness by finding out a bit more about some of the treatments or medication I have been given. Remember that the brain you had before you got ill is still functioning; you do not need to check it in at the hospital door. While we don't want to frighten ourselves with a little knowledge or incorrect information, it is good to know what is happening to your body. Whether this is just reading the leaflets that come with the medication, looking up information on the internet, reading leaflets available in the hospital or reading books, informing ourselves is a good thing.

I am not suggesting that you act on this information without consultation with the doctors, but you can discuss information you find or worries you have. I have done this with my own treatment and always found the doctors willing to answer my queries. It has helped me understand better what is going on and kept me from feeling so frightened. If you do not feel able to do this, perhaps there is a family member or a friend that will act as your buddy in this role.

The medical system is there to help us. In dealing with it we should feel reassured, not more confused or lost. Whether we are dealing with consultants, our GP, nurses or the various technicians we meet, we need to feel confident enough to ask questions, to query what is being done for us and to ask for time to think about something if we feel that is necessary.

I used to feel that these were important people with busy jobs and that I couldn't hold them up with what might seem to be silly queries. However, over the years I have realised that their busy jobs involve my health and that their importance lies in the skills they apply to my illness. I need to work with them to help improve my quality of life within the boundaries of the illness. I am doing them and myself no favours by keeping quiet. I have also found that I follow their directions more carefully when I understand why I am doing what they ask. My motto is to try to be part of the team that is keeping me okay. As I said at the beginning, attending the hospital is still a stressful experience but I can take responsibility and try to minimise this stress as much as possible.

Thirteenth-century Persian poet Sa'di said, 'A traveller without knowledge is a bird without wings', and this holds much truth for those of us who are journeying through illness.

MAIN POINTS

Prepare the questions you want to ask the doctors in advance of your appointment.

Read up on your illness; familiarise yourself with the terms used.

Don't be afraid to say that you don't understand.

Bring somebody to appointments with you to be that extra ear.

Give the doctors the information they need to help you.

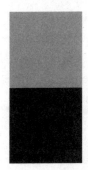

chapter 3

Asking for and Accepting Help

We do not always have to look ill to be ill. There are many people that we meet every day that are silently suffering and trying to get on with their lives.

None of us want to be looked at by people who pity us or who thank God that they aren't us. I don't want to be defined by my illness or pitied for it. However, it has been my experience that if someone knows you are ill they might just make that allowance or offer that bit of help that could make your day bearable.

There are the days that we can be feeling foul, just about struggling to get by, but because we look okay too much is expected from us. We are all inclined to take people at face value: if people look well they are well.

Yet sometimes we are not well, we are not okay. The illness inside us affects how we relate to others, how we handle situations, in fact, how we interact with the rest of the world. The outward mask at these times doesn't reflect our inner self.

Many illnesses have their good days and their bad days; days when we feel we can handle daily life and days when we want to crawl back under the duvet and pray for sleep to return. Perhaps some days our daily routine is just too much. We are, I think, reluctant to tell people what is wrong with us in case they think we are courting sympathy or trying to duck out of our fair share of work.

So what can we do if our illness is invisible to the outside world? We need to work out a strategy for ourselves, one that helps us cope yet doesn't leave us feeling uncomfortable or compromised in our own eyes. On days that I was too unwell to perform simple tasks I felt very down. I wanted help from people but expected them to realise what I needed without my asking. Then I would get cross with others and feel sorry for myself. I was resentful of what I perceived as people's uncaring attitude. This mix of feelings wasn't doing me any good; it definitely wasn't helping my health.

When I thought about it I realised I wanted people to be mind readers. I expected them to know what was going on with me without any clues. This didn't work – even the best detectives would have failed! The solution was simple: I had to tell them what I wanted and how I was feeling; to say straight out, 'I'm not feeling too good today, you'll have to excuse me/help me'.

This can be a very hard step to take. I found it easier when I imagined it from the other side of the fence: if I had a friend, family member or work colleague who was suffering I would like to know – not to pity them, but to understand what was going on for them. It is alright for people to make allowances for us and I, for one, would prefer to know that a person was acting strangely because of the way they were feeling rather than because of something I did. We like our independence but we should be careful not to mistake care and compassion from others as pity.

Of course, this works with those we know but what about the strangers we meet every day. They see a relatively healthy fit person and have no reason to suspect we are ill. Someone can suffer from severe pains and aches that aren't outwardly visible. Therefore strangers do not realise they are ill. Honesty is the best policy I have learnt. If somebody asks me to do something the best thing is just to say straight out, 'Sorry, but I can't because I have ...'. Generally, people will be glad you told them. We have no reason to be ashamed if we are ill. It is a fact of life that some of us get sick. We didn't ask for illness but there it is and we need to adapt to live with it. There are things we cannot do any more, but hopefully there are also lots of things we can still do and enjoy.

Just because an illness and its effects are invisible doesn't mean it's not there. We have to be honest with ourselves and realise that our reserves of energy are precious and need to be kept for the positive things in our life. We need to listen to our body – it knows what it can and cannot do.

HIDDEN PAIN
A leg weighed down by plaster,
an arm captured by a sling.
These bring cries of sympathy,
questions gently asked

'What can I do to help
to ease the problem?'
But what of the pain
buried deep within bones.
Pain that gives little rest
and drains my strength.
Invisible pain
leaves the sufferer to
bear it alone.

I wrote this poem when I was feeling down, feeling that nobody knew what I was going through. I also wrote it for others who are suffering silently. Now, years on, I know what I need to do: I need to give invisible pain a voice, not a whining or a fearful voice but a strong, confident voice. I need to explain to others what is happening for me. I don't have to do it all alone.

Accepting the help of family and friends, of those we work with or of strangers that we meet is no shame. It took me some time to come to this conclusion. In refusing the help we are locking these people out, people that love us; we are saying to them we can manage without them.

I came to enjoy the small and big acts of kindness and learned to take them for what they were and not see them as condescending pity from those healthier than me and therefore, by my definition, superior to me. I appreciate the kindness of the person who quietly left a small gift at my front door on my bad days; the neighbour who happily minded my child when I couldn't; the many who cooked for me, ironed for me, prayed for me. These people showed their care in so many small and big ways. I appreciate the kindness of my family who minded me and took on what I could not do. They all wrapped me in their care. The important part was how I received it. Once I looked on all this help as a good thing I felt overwhelmed by the kindness and love of others. It is a step on the road to healing.

In *The Prophet*, Kahlil Gibran talks of the giving and receiving of help. To the receivers he says:

> And you receivers – and you
> are all receivers –
> assume no weight of gratitude,
> lest you lay a yoke upon
> yourself and
> upon him who gives.

Rather rise together with the
giver on
his gifts as on wings;
For to be overmindful of your
debt
is to doubt his generosity who
has the
free-hearted earth for mother
and God
for Father.

MAIN POINTS

Be prepared to tell others when
you are not feeling up to a task.

Don't be ashamed of being ill.

Accept the compassion of others
graciously.

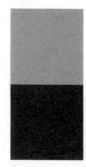

chapter 4

Caring Support and Supporting the Carers

At the time I first fell ill I had a very full and satisfying life. I worked full time in the home looking after my family. My youngest son was then seven years old and being with him and all that is entailed in raising a young child was a large part of my daily life. I was also very involved in volunteer work with my local community and parish. I was in my forties, feeling fulfilled in my life and enjoying it thoroughly.

Illness brought many changes to this lifestyle. The acute part of my illness lasted for a year. At the beginning my health wasn't too bad and I was able to maintain a normal life to a certain degree, but as the year progressed this became very difficult.

I was no longer able to do things that I had taken for granted. I got to a stage where I was dependent on others to do many things for me. It isn't until you cannot continue with the daily tasks that you realise how much you took for granted your ability to do them. I am a very independent person and also have a tendency to think that others cannot do the task as well as I can. I found it very hard to relinquish the reins to others. Yet I did have to finally admit that I needed to do so – for my own sake as well as for those around me who loved and worried about me.

I know that when I was ill those who loved me felt very helpless – they were on the outside looking in. The medical team seem to be the people you rely on, and family and friends are not sure what they can do to help. In a crisis situation people need to feel that they can contribute in some way; if they are worried or scared they need activity and involvement to help them feel they have some control over the situation.

In Chapter 3, I talked about asking for and accepting help and why this is so important for us. However, it is also important for our families and friends, and can be a support for them during this very difficult time. It may sound incongruous – supporting our families even though it is us who are ill and dependent on them – but there is much we can do to help those that look after us on a daily basis. Looking after someone in the long term can be extremely exhausting. We need to be aware that carers haven't got a bottomless pit of reserves to call upon and they too need to be cared for.

When I was ill, my husband was put under great strain. On top of the emotional strain, there was the practical difficulty of taking on the many tasks that I had previously taken responsibility for. In the beginning I was reluctant to take help from friends and neighbours with many of the ordinary tasks that have to be done each day. I wanted to prove that I could still get on with them, to show everybody that I could manage. But I couldn't manage and there was nothing I could do to alter the fact that this extra responsibility for many jobs around the home and with the children fell to my husband. When I was in hospital he was running in each day to see me; on top of this he was trying to feed the family, deal with the housework and go to work himself. When I was home and going through chemotherapy and radiotherapy treatment, he was trying to take on what I couldn't do.

Eventually, I realised that this couldn't go on in the long term and that the only way I could help my husband was by letting others help when they offered. The final breakthrough came when I decided to let a friend clean my sitting room. This may not sound like much, but for me it was a big step. The room was getting more and more untidy and a good friend had asked me many times what she could do to help. My husband knew that the room was getting me down and was trying to find time to give it a good spring clean. When I think back I am ashamed to admit that I was nearly prepared to let him just to keep up the pretence. But one day when my friend asked I said 'Yes' and up she arrived with rubber gloves and duster and set to. This was a moment of revelation for me: I realised that she didn't think any less of me for admitting that I couldn't do this job and I think she got joy from being able to help me. Even more important, I didn't further overburden my husband by letting him take on this task just so I could 'save face'.

When a loved one is caring for us we need to be aware of all they are doing. They are looking after us while taking on our jobs and continuing with their own. We need to show our appreciation for what they are doing. Of course, they do what they do out of love and are not looking for thanks or reward, but why not say 'Thank you' and tell them how much it means to us.

We also need to remember that they need to recharge their batteries too. We need to make sure that they get time to themselves and allow them to have their bad days. Just because we are sick we shouldn't take away their permission to be out of sorts with us. As much as possible, we need to maintain and enjoy the 'normal' life we shared with them before the illness.

MAIN POINTS

Do not expect your primary carer to take on all that entails single-handedly.

Tell those who care for you how much you appreciate them.

Allow them to be down, to be cross with you, to treat you as they always did.

Make sure that they get a break and a chance to recharge their batteries.

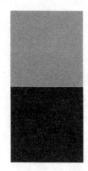

chapter 5

Talking to Children: What Do You Say?

My children were aged twenty, seventeen and seven when I first found out I was seriously ill. Talking to them about it and deciding what to tell them was extremely difficult.

What I am saying here comes from my experience as a parent but I feel that it is applicable to any significant adult/child relationship. You might not have young children of your own but most people have some contact with young children and when we get ill it affects their lives. You might have grandchildren, nieces or nephews, or younger brothers or sisters; you may work closely with children.

If you play a significant role in a child's life, telling them that you are very ill is going to upset and confuse them. I think it is necessary to give some thought to the way you will approach the topic with the child.

The age of the child must be taken into consideration. The approach I took with my twenty year old, an adult, and with my seventeen year old, in the later stages of adolescence, was quite different to the approach I took with my seven year old.

I must be honest and say that I didn't handle it well in the initial stages. The beginning of my illness fell around Christmas and this gave me a good reason to defer talking to my youngest. After Christmas the time for going into hospital was fast approaching and I still hadn't said anything. He found me crying one day and then I had to talk. I wish I had done it differently.

Children are clever and very observant. They have an antenna for when something is not right and I feel that you are better off coming clean in the first place. They also have very active imaginations and what they imagine can be much worse than the reality.

I think it is important, though, to match the amount and level of information given to the child's age. In most cases young children don't want too much detail. We handled the situation by letting our youngest know what was happening, when I would be going into hospital and what was wrong with me. We tried not to be secretive about it but not to dramatise it too much either.

Don't be surprised if they get angry with you. I know I was frightened by all that was going on, so it isn't surprising that a child will be frightened too and express this fear through anger. If they are of school-going age it can be a good idea to let the school and the child's teacher know what is happening at home. This helps the teacher understand why the child might be acting out of character and will allow them to be more understanding.

I suppose most of what I have said so far is in relation to a parent and child situation, but I think a lot of it can apply in other adult/child relationships. A child often has a very close relationship with a grandparent, or an aunt or uncle. They will notice if their parents are upset about an illness in the family. In this situation, though they are not dealing with the day-to-day effects of the illness, it is still important to let the child know what is going on. When my mother and sister fell ill, I let the boys know and explained to them what was happening. Needless to say, if you are not related to the child it would be vital to discuss with the parents how they feel you should handle the situation.

There are many ways to help children understand what is going on and we all have to find a way that suits them, and us, best. You can sit the child down and explain to them simply and briefly what is happening and assure them that you will keep them informed of what is going on. Reading them an appropriate book can introduce the illness to them gently. (Always read a book like this first so that you know what is in it and are happy with the content.) In the case of it being your own child they could accompany you on a hospital visit. Seeing where you go should help remove some of the mystery around the situation and make it less frightening.

When a parent is ill, the child's life is turned upside down. When I had to have chemotherapy I was quite weak. All my sons helped me in different ways. There are many little things even the youngest child can do for you.

You know the personality of the children you are dealing with best and are therefore the most suitable person to judge the right approach to take with them. What I have said here is just from my own experience and I have only touched briefly on the subject, but I hope you will find some help in what I have said.

We should never underestimate children and their ability to deal with a difficult situation. I found my children a great support and joy to me in my illness and I know that they were glad to hear that their help made a difference to me.

I read what I felt was a very wise insight on children. I don't remember the author; it was just something that I identified with and wrote down and kept.

> While we try to teach our children all about life, our children teach us what life is all about.

Plan what you are going to say to a child before you start talking to them.

Be honest with them but don't overload them with information.

Let them help you: it can make them feel part of what is happening. Let them know how much you value that help.

Let their school know what is going on.

chapter 6

Listen to your Body

For at least six months before I fell ill I was not feeling fully myself. It is hard to describe exactly what was wrong but I felt a coldness inside that I couldn't seem to find a reason for. In hindsight there were also other signs. I felt weary a lot of the time and did not have my usual enthusiasm for life. It is easy now to say that something was wrong but at the time I put it down to the ordinary stresses and strains of life.

These days, life for many of us is very busy. A friend remarked to me the other day that somebody must be stealing time; that the days and weeks couldn't be going as fast as they seemed to be. Indeed, the week seems just to have begun and we have arrived at the weekend once again. We are left with the list of tasks we thought we could accomplish and instead of crossing items off the list we seem to have added more!

It is perhaps too simple to suggest that we try not to go so fast. For a lot of us, stepping off the merry-go-round of daily tasks is easier said than done. Yet if we want to achieve some balance in the way we live our life we need to find a way to manage all the stuff that comes at us on a daily basis. I found that when I was diagnosed with cancer that decision was forced on me, my way of life had to be altered. For those of us who get this warning but still manage to recover and go on with our lives, it is vital that we remember where we have come from and try to do all that is in our power not to end up back there again.

Our body is a strange and complex thing. It serves us well and takes a lot of punishment. The body is also a barometer of how we are; in its own way it talks to us and we need to listen to what it has to say.

We all know that feeling that comes at a time of over-indulgence, when we eat the wrong foods or too much food; when we don't get enough sleep or rest. Our body quickly lets us know that we are mistreating it. Similarly, if a part of our body is not working properly and if something is attacking it, we also know. At a very simple level, when we get a cold or flu the symptoms are very obvious and we know there is something alien in our system. If we try to ignore this and go on with our normal lives we find that we soon have to give in and allow our body time to recover. We can fool others that we are okay, but we cannot fool our body. It will go on strike and refuse to function until we give it the care it deserves.

It is now six years on from the time when I was acutely ill yet I still think that I need to be aware of the consequences that this illness has had on my physical well-being. In the year after my illness I resented people saying to me that I needed to take it easy, not to be rushing to do everything all at once. I felt that I was cured and that normal life could resume. However, as time went on I learned that this was not the case. There were adjustments that I needed to make and, in the end, this helped me return more quickly to what I wanted to do.

When I truly listen to my body I know that I do not have the ability to do all that I did before. I have had to reassess what is really important in my life; I have to pace myself and prioritise what is most valuable to me.

I also need to be aware when my body is not feeling up to scratch and try to work out why. This does not mean having an unhealthy preoccupation with every ache and pain that comes my way. For me it is a positive action. At the beginning I used to fear every unknown pain. I would build up a scenario around it and before I knew it I would have myself dead and buried. I had forgotten that even before I got sick there were days that I would have unexplained pains, but back then I had no history that made me fear them. Marcel Proust said:

> it is in moments of illness that we are compelled to recognise that we live not alone but chained to a creature of a different kingdom, whole worlds apart, who has no knowledge of us and by whom it is impossible to make ourselves understood: our body.

It may be true that our body has no knowledge of us but I feel a new need to have knowledge of my body; to know for myself what is good for it and what isn't, to take note of when it runs well and when I feel that we are fighting against each other. I also need to become aware of when it needs me to get help for it. I feel now that I have come to a point in my life where I feel happier finding out what the unexplained pain is. I have found that most of the time it is nothing but I know that I am better off with the explanation, whatever that may be.

When I am well and getting on with everyday life I am not aware of my body. It is only when it lets me down, when sickness interferes with what I want to do, that I become acutely aware of it and my dependence on it. Becoming tuned to its needs is the only wise course to adopt and I believe one that will give me a better quality of life.

Don't ignore the physical signs that say your body is not functioning as it should.

Accept that you cannot do everything; prioritise.

If something is wrong, it is better to find out; ignoring it doesn't make it go away.

Become friends with your body; get to know it and what it needs.

chapter 7

The Unexpected Response: How Others React

When I got ill I didn't feel that I became my illness. I did have difficulty adjusting to the changes it brought and it did have a bearing on how I lived, but at no time did I feel that it defined me. I had cancer, but I still enjoyed doing the things that I always had done. None of that had changed. My illness changed my outward appearance: certain medicine made me put on weight; I lost my hair and had to wear a wig, but I still thought of myself as me. I didn't suddenly see myself as the cancer patient. However, it seemed that is how some people saw me.

I have learnt through my illness to expect the unexpected. People I didn't know very well came to me with offers of help and some I thought I knew well avoided me. I told myself that this was some lack in them and not in me, but it still hurt. One day I was out with my husband and we met a person we knew from the neighbourhood. Now this was a good and kind man, but when he turned to Paul and asked, 'How is Catherine? Is she doing okay?', I felt shattered and was near to tears. Had I suddenly become invisible? Did he think that illness had deprived me of the power of speech? Paul stuttered an answer and we walked on. I realised, on reflection, that this man had not intended to be cruel; it was just that he didn't know how to talk to me.

I think that we are all guilty of this at some time. It is the rare person that always knows the right thing to say. I wondered if I had been guilty of the same awkwardness and insensitivity in the past. It can be difficult to deal with someone who is ill, especially someone who has a life-threatening illness. We are afraid we might say the wrong thing. Maybe we feel uncomfortable around such a definite example of our own immortality.

Let me make a simple point here that we sometimes forget: sick people are no different from healthy people except that their bodies are not working properly, whether that is for a set length of time or for always: that is the only difference.

When I was sick I was still capable of laughing or crying. I still wanted to go out, still wanted to do all the things I had done before; the only difference was I wasn't quite able to do them to the same extent. More than anything, I wanted people to treat me the same as they had always done.

When we are sick we are isolated from the real world in so many ways that we long for those around us, our family and friends, to treat us as normal. We long to be our old selves and to have others treat us as such. We should feel free to say this to those around us, whether they be family, friends, neighbours or work colleagues. There is nothing wrong in saying to them that you want them to remember the real you, not the one who looks grotty and frail, and that you want them to treat you as they always did. They are our link with reality; they are the ones who help us remember who we are and who we will be again. Tell them that the best compliment they can pay is to assume that we are still able to deal with the day-to-day stuff of ordinary life.

I remember my eldest son having an argument with me one day when I was feeling particularly weak. I can't remember what it was about, just one of those everyday things. At first I thought to myself, 'How can he treat me like this? Doesn't he know that I'm not able for it?' Afterwards, however, I thought that he had payed me the greatest compliment: he had treated me like his mother; he hadn't sidelined me because I was ill and tiptoed around me. I knew then that this is what I wanted from everybody.

As a seriously ill person I think we should be thankful for all those family and friends who are not handling us with kid gloves.

I was grateful to those who didn't change the subject when I entered the room. I was grateful to friends who still asked if I fancied a night out. All this helped me to avoid the trap of feeling too sorry for myself. I gladly grabbed the offer with both hands. Maybe I wasn't always up to my usual standards and sometimes I had to go home early, but I was willing to give it a shot and really appreciated their willingness to be with me on my terms.

Your illness does not define who you are, it is just another part of the whole you.

Remember that people sometimes find it difficult to deal comfortably with someone who is very ill.

It is alright to ask family and friends to treat you as they always have done.

coping with serious illness

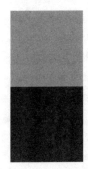

chapter 8

A Spiritual Dimension

Getting cancer at forty-five was not expected and not easily accepted either. I had a family, a busy and productive life, and this was not supposed to happen. I know that everybody deals with adversity in their own way. For me I knew that I had a fight on my hands. Pretending I wasn't ill wouldn't make the illness go away. There was going to be much pain and discomfort to be got through if I had any hope of coming out the other side. My determination, the doctor's medical expertise, help and encouragement from family and friends, were just some of the tools available to me. Another essential tool was my faith.

My faith had never really been tested up to the moment of my diagnosis. There had been no major tragedy in my life. My father died when I was twenty and that was a great sadness. To this day I still feel his loss. I feel that he died when we were moving out of the difficult arguing stage and becoming friends. However, though I mourn him, and at the time questioned the reason for his death, it was not a totally unexpected happening. Since that time, even though there have been ups and downs in life, I took them as they came. None of us can expect to be happy all the time.

Faith or the spiritual dimension in life is a very personal thing. For some people I know it is very hard to reconcile something seriously bad happening with the idea of a loving God. For me, though, my faith was an essential component during my illness from which I drew strength in the dark days. That is not to say that from the first moment of diagnosis I felt peaceful, calm and supported by an inner belief. Far from it! Ultimately, however, this experience turned me more towards my God than away from him.

I am not trying to suggest that those who do not have a belief in a deity have no spiritual strength to draw upon. When you are ill, medicine isn't the only thing that helps. While the medicine is working on your body, your soul too needs its own medicine. Acts of kindness and care from others go so far to provide this medicine for the soul. These do not have to be big gestures and often their benefit far outweighs the amount of effort that someone feels they put into them.

I had very many such kindnesses throughout the time I was seriously ill. One friend would often take me on a drive out to the country for a walk and coffee. Driving along seeing the sunlight playing on the trees, or walking in the warm sunshine gave me strength. Another friend read somewhere that the colour red was supposed to give strength and she arrived at my door with a red cardigan for me to wear when I was feeling weak. When I wrapped it around me I could feel her good wishes coming to me. Yet another friend left a small gift in my porch when she knew I was going for a chemotherapy session. Arriving home and finding this brought joy to me at a time I was feeling truly awful. Others cooked meals and bread for the family. They arrived at the door quietly with their offering, not realising that there was far more than just a practical support to their kindnesses. Another friend collected my youngest from school each day when I wasn't able. It meant so much to be able to rest, safe in the knowledge that he was happy and cared for.

All these kindnesses and many more that I haven't mentioned lifted my spirits when I needed it most and left me basking in the warmth of their love and care. This to me was their spirituality at work even though they may not have considered it as such.

Nature can also soothe a sore spirit. While I was in the middle of my chemotherapy we took a short family break to Dingle in Kerry. On the Friday morning before our return home we went for a walk along the shore. I sat on a rock listening to the sounds of the seabirds, looking at the sun sparkling on the water and feeling it warm on my back. I stored up that memory for the following Friday, when I knew I would be sitting in the hospital going through another bout of chemotherapy. As I sat in the hospital ward I closed my eyes and was back on that sunny seashore. That for me was a spiritual experience and one that helped me endure what was happening.

We can also draw solace from poetry and music. We all have something in our lives that comforts and soothes us and that we can draw on when we are most in need. Poetry can bring us the wisdom of others and can speak to our situation. A poem that most of us learned at school, William Wordsworth's 'The Daffodils', talks of this:

> When oft on my couch I lie
> in vacant or in pensive mood,
> they flash upon that inward eye
> which is the bliss of solitude;
> and then my heart with pleasure fills
> and dances with the daffodils.

Just because this poem is so familiar, should not minimise its truth for us.

It would be arrogant of me to suggest to anybody where they might find spiritual solace in the face of serious illness. Whether it comes from a belief in a deity, from nature, from poetry, from music or from a combination of all these sources is, I believe, an individual's own choice. I can only share with you my own experience. I found it essential to medicate my spirit just as my body was being medicated. I needed this to keep going in the face of all that was happening and to give me strength for what might be to come. It is nearly impossible in the darkness of despair sometimes to see any chink of light and anything that gets us through is a tool to be used and appreciated.

I found these verses from 'Desiderata' very comforting when I was feeling lost and questioning all that was happening to me:

> You are a child of the universe,
> no less than the trees and the
> stars;
> you have a right to be here.
> And whether or not it is clear
> to you,
> no doubt the universe is
> unfolding as it should.
> Therefore be at peace with God,
> whatever you conceive Him to
> be,
> and whatever your labors and
> aspirations,
> in the noisy confusion of life
> keep peace with your soul.
> With all its sham, drudgery,
> and broken dreams,
> it is still a beautiful world.

coping with serious illness

Be cheerful.
Strive to be happy.

(Max Ehrmann, 'Desiderata')

MAIN POINTS

Don't underestimate the benefit you can get from the spiritual in your fight against illness.

Remember where you received solace in difficult times before you were ill and try to tap into those things now.

Little gestures can mean such a lot to the receiver, often more than the giver realises.

chapter 9

Feeling Guilty: Did I Do Something to Cause my Illness?

When you are diagnosed with serious illness the last thing you expect to feel is guilty. At first you feel the shock that this has happened to you and then the fear of what will happen in the future kicks in. Yet when I started to feel guilty this emotion was totally unexpected and I didn't quite know how to handle it.

A friend had given me a book called *Love, Medicine and Miracles* by Dr Bernie Siegel. She thought it would help me. The theme of the book was how seriously ill people could take control of their illness. It talked of the different reactions people have to an initial diagnosis and then to the fight ahead of them. It also raised the question of how some people fell ill while others who might seem more likely to contract illness didn't. It talked a lot about our frame of mind when we first fall ill.

Maybe I picked up the wrong message, but the author definitely seemed to be saying that when your life isn't going too well your immune system may not be working correctly and that is the time that illness can take over. Whether it be justified or not, I began to question if there was something I did that caused my illness. I thought about it a lot; going over in my head how I felt around the time I was first diagnosed. Had I been down, allowing negative emotions free rein? Had I brought all this on myself? These thoughts went round and round in my head until I didn't know what to think.

Serious life-threatening illness is devastating. Your body is sick and weak when you most need to marshal your resources to resist the illness. Having to also take on board the question of whether you had something to do with this awful thing that has come your way can be one burden too many.

Why do we get seriously ill? There are many answers to this question and I, as a layperson, am not fully qualified to answer it. No illness is simple; the issues are many and complex. Just to look at it very superficially, I suppose my immediate thoughts would be that an illness can come from a predisposition in your family; perhaps lifestyle can contribute to it also. When we are ill, our attitudes to the illness can be varied: some people want to hide it and pretend it hasn't happened; others see it as something to be conquered. We all have our individual reactions and all are valid.

We can all do without also having to deal with a feeling of guilt. Once the illness has occurred there is nothing to be gained by wasting our limited energy blaming ourselves. All the hours we spend picking through the past are not going to change anything. We need to keep strong for the journey ahead.

I have recently read a book called *The Power of Now* by Eckhart Tolle and I wish I had read it years ago. The main theme of the book is that your life is happening now – not in the past or in the future. We can learn from the past and plan for the future, but we cannot live in either. We have to live now.

I was, and to some extent still am, the sort of person that worries about things – often things that never happen. We all have certain lifestyles when we fall ill, we may wonder what part that lifestyle played in bringing us to where we are now, but the only reason we should dwell on this is if we are looking for ways to change. Life is hard enough without wasting time beating ourselves up over what we cannot change.

Guilt in itself has no value. When I first read my friend's book, I felt angry and annoyed – I had got the damned cancer and now here was somebody trying to blame me for it. When I calmed down, however, and re-read the book, I realised that this was not what the author was saying. Dr Siegel says that although blaming oneself is not ideal, 'this attitude is not entirely destructive, for it often leads to a more realistic sense of participation in the onset of disease'. Even if I did now feel some guilt about my illness, I could learn from it and try to do all I could to make sure it didn't happen again, thereby reducing my sense of powerlessness and helping me plan to be less vulnerable in the future.

An important part of any illness is retaining our feeling that we still have power over what is happening to us. We can also harness that power to deal with what is going on for us. If studying all the emotions we feel, including ones of guilt, allows us to do this then it is worth examining them and working with them to help ourselves. We need to do this gently, thoughtfully and with compassion for ourselves.

I have lately come across a poem written by cartoonist Michael Leunig in his book *Short Notes from the Long History of Happiness*. I think it is apt for us to remember when we are trying to examine the whys and wherefore of where we are in our life:

> God help us to live slowly:
> To move simply:
> To look softly:
> To allow emptiness:
> To let the heart create for us.
> Amen.

Try not to revisit the past unless it is to learn from it. Then by all means visit but don't live there.

Don't beat yourself up over what you cannot change.

Realise that you haven't lost all power over your life just because you are ill – use the power you have to your benefit.

chapter 10

Shared Experience:
The Value of
Talking to Others

There are many old proverbs that
recommend the value of talking to others
when we feel down or in trouble – 'A trouble
shared is a trouble halved', for example. We
quote them so often that we can miss the
fact that they might offer valuable insight.

In day-to-day life, we are not inclined to
want to burden others with our problems. If
asked how we are, we give the pat answer
and move on. Most of us have family and
friends that we go to when we are feeling
down or want to discuss a thorny issue.
However, when we are seriously ill, it can
also help to talk to somebody who is going
through the same experience as you.

When I was seriously ill I found that it
lightened the load a little to talk to
somebody that was in the same boat. I am
not suggesting that to talk about what you

are going through takes away the pain or the suffering. Yet for me to know that there is someone to talk to who knows exactly what I am on about helps a little.

When I went to the hospital for regular chemotherapy or radiotherapy sessions I nearly always got chatting with the person sitting beside me. Sometimes we would talk about what was going on for us and it could be a relief to hear that a symptom you had and were really worried about was happening to someone else too. There were days when I was feeling really down and sorry for myself, yet when I heard others' stories I came away thinking I wasn't too bad and that I wasn't the only one going through this.

While my cancer is always with me and will always colour the rest of my life, the acute stage did have a beginning, a middle and an end. The beginning occurred with my diagnosis and operation. The middle was the intense period of chemotherapy and radiotherapy treatment. This lasted for nine months and when it ended I felt lost and more than a bit scared. While having treatment I felt at least I was doing something, dealing with my illness. Much as

I longed for the treatment to stop, when it did I wasn't sure what would come next. Was I now to get on with my life? How would I do this? My body was different, my level of energy definitely different – how was I to handle it all?

Then somebody told me of a course that was supposed to help people deal with illness and recommended that I give it a try. I wasn't sure about this; I just wanted to put the last nine months behind me and get on with the rest of my life. I wondered if joining a group to talk about all that had happened for me would be just wallowing in self-pity. I debated with myself as to the pros and cons of attending the course. On reflection I realised that it could help to answer some of those questions I had asked myself and this in turn would help me to move on with the next stage of my life.

I attended the course and over the weeks I got to know the other people very well. We were all there with different illnesses but one common goal: we wanted to learn how to live our lives within the boundaries of the illness we had. I learned a lot from the group, safely guided by a facilitator. We got great support from each other, talking about our fears and our hopes; about other people's reactions to us and what they expected from us; about our good days and bad days.

For me, the course was a stepping-stone on a journey back to the real world. For some, their illnesses would have a more long-term and invasive impact on their futures but they too felt as if they had been given support for their fight. On the last day one of the participants, who had touched us all with her story, brought a gift for each of us. The gift was a candle holder in the shape of a silver coffee cup and saucer. We were all very moved by this gesture and to this day that cup sits in my kitchen. I often light it and remember the experiences that I shared with that group. I am thankful that I overcame my reluctance and took the decision to attend the course.

There are many organisations and groups out there offering to support those with serious illness. Many of the people involved have already been through what is happening to us. These groups may not suit everybody but it is worth giving them a try. This is a difficult battle we are fighting and if there is something that might help, even if only a little, why not give it a shot? None of these organisations is looking for a lifetime commitment from us; they are there to help and might just be another tool we can use.

MAIN POINTS

Talking to someone who has had or is having a similar experience can be supportive.

It is worth trying out the different tools available to get help.

Joining a support group is a way to talk to others in a protected environment.

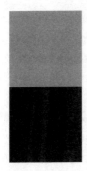

chapter 11

Treasuring the Small Things

Remember that song from *The Sound of Music* ...

> When the dog bites, when the
> bee stings,
> when I'm feeling sad,
> I simply remember my favourite
> things
> and then I don't feel so bad.

This is what I need to do sometimes when it all gets too much – I look to the everyday small things that I get pleasure from, or have got pleasure from in the past. This may sound a very simplistic thing to say to somebody who is in great pain and labouring under all the unpleasantness that serious illness brings, but I truly find that when despair is great, it is sometimes the simple things that pull us through.

When my first child was small, going for a walk with him was an adventure in itself. Before he was born I would go to the local shops (a journey on foot of little over five minutes), buy what I needed and head back home oblivious to most of what was around me. With him in tow, the journey was very different. We stopped to look at the daisies and dandelions in the grass. The birds were pointed out and gazed at ... at length. Trucks, fire brigades and any big four-wheeled vehicles were truly amazing. Without sounding sentimental, I truly rediscovered ordinary, everyday items through his eyes.

Some years later, when I was unwell, I was taken back to that time. The short walk to the shop became a marathon and my thoughts returned to those early walks with my son. Everything I was used to doing at a fast past had to be taken slowly to make it possible at all, which was very frustrating. Frequent stops to catch my breath forced me to look around and, despite myself, I started to see some of the beauty in everyday things and was nourished by them.

We all have our list of our own favourite things that are very personal to us. In most cases they are not the big events, but just things that we savour and that can renew our spirits when they're low. When 'the dog bites, when the bee stings' I need something to anesthetise the pain, and that is when I dip into my treasure trove of favourite things.

I don't know what your personal experience of serious illness is. I don't know if it is something that will last for a set period or whether it is something that is going to be with you always. I realise that by thinking or doing something nice our pain or sickness does not disappear, but if we can find something that lifts us maybe we can mentally step out for a time. Then perhaps we can come back a little refreshed, a little nourished and a little stronger for the battle ahead.

At a time when I was frequently confined to bed, a friend gave me a little pot of miniature daffodils. As they sat on my bedside table, the vibrancy and energy of those small yellow flowers gave me much pleasure. I could list here many things that sustained me, but that would be my list and

I am sure you would have more fun putting together one of your own.

I found it really worthwhile getting hold of a small notebook, one that can be easily carried around in a pocket, and writing down the small things that gave me pleasure as they occurred. Then when you are feeling too bad to even think, your notebook can be a memory aid to help lift you for that precious few minutes.

I was listening to the radio just the other day and I heard a song being played that I immediately took a liking to. Knowing that my memory is so bad and that I wouldn't remember it I quickly grabbed paper and pen to write down the name of the band and the line that appealed to me. I find myself doing this often now and recording things that please me and storing them up for the days that I might need them.

The line of the song that I scribbled down that day was by an Irish group named BellX1:

> I want to be near you and bathe
> in your light
> and toast marshmallows on a
> cold dark night.

This is such a simple concept, yet for me it conjured up visions of comfort and togetherness. I added it to my list. Another person may be totally unmoved by this and that is why I feel that each person's list will be so individual and totally for them. When you are ill anything that helps you bear what is going on and bring you spiritual and emotional nourishment can only be good for you.

My favourite things are part of my toolbox for the hard times. Have fun filling yours with your favourite things.

EVERYTHING IS GOING TO BE ALRIGHT
How should I not be glad to contemplate
the clouds clearing beyond the dormer window
and a high tide reflected on the ceiling?
There will be dying, there will be dying,
but there is no need to go into that.
The poems flow from the hand unbidden

and the hidden source is the
watchful heart.
The sun rises despite everything
and the far cities are beautiful
and bright.
I lie here in a riot of sunlight
watching the day break and the
clouds flying.
Everything is going to be
alright.

(Derek Mahon)

MAIN POINTS

When the suffering is really bad
it can be the small pleasures that
give us a lift.

Try to use the enforced slowing
of the pace of your life to see
everything through fresh eyes.

Compile your list of favourite
things, the ones that give you a
lift, in a small notebook and call
on it when you are low.

chapter 12

Survival Strategies

When I was ill, the acute stage lasted for about a year. As for the subsequent stage, well that, I suppose, will be with me forever. Through all of this I felt and still feel it necessary to have my survival strategies. These helped me over the worst bits and gave me the energy and courage to pick myself up and get going again.

I had many, ranging from long-term changes to my lifestyle to the more fire-brigade varieties, the ones that were short term and indeed could only be indulged in for a short length of time. You may already have strategies of your own to help you along but let me introduce you to some of mine so you will get an idea of what I mean.

I had a course of chemotherapy every third Friday. I had twelve sessions in all. In the beginning my husband came with me for the full day but as time went on and as I got used to the routine I went on my own, but he always arrived for the end of the session to accompany me home. On route, we would stop at the 'chemo café', as we christened it, for a coffee and some type of sticky sugary confection. I would enjoy this thoroughly before the inevitable nausea set in. I'm sure that the lovely coffee shop wouldn't have appreciated our nickname for it, but I hope it would have been happy with the support these visits gave me.

Light-hearted programmes on the TV that made me laugh and distracted my mind for a while were also a great way of filling in the time when I didn't even have the energy to hold a book. The family bought me a small TV for the bedroom and it definitely was a good friend at these times.

I learned the valuable lesson of asking for help. As I said earlier, in the beginning I thought I could do it all on my own; I felt I was giving into the illness if I couldn't keep going as usual. However, I learned very quickly to appreciate the help that was being offered with such kindness and to accept it graciously. All the help that was offered so willingly gave me a long-term belief in the kindness of others.

I also learned to decide quickly what tasks had to be done and what ones could be shelved. In fact, some of them I shelved forever. I discovered that the world wasn't going to fall apart if I didn't iron every item in the laundry basket. Also that the house would look just as good with a lick and a promise as an in-depth clean.

A wise person told me that I should avoid those people that would bring me down. I needed to keep a positive frame of mind and surround myself with people who believed that this was only a blip in my life – a major blip – but one that could be overcome. Therefore, I learned to know those that would help and those, however well-meaning, who would leave me feeling worse rather than better. My energy was scarce and I needed to guard it carefully.

It is difficult to take a long holiday when you are tied to a hospital schedule, but short breaks are possible. I returned from them refreshed and ready for the next step. They were also precious time spent with family and friends. Sometimes just a day out to walk in the country or to visit an art gallery was enough to lift my spirits.

I have always loved poetry, especially that of Robert Frost. Sometimes a poet can express so well what I am thinking and their words nourish and soothe. I like to keep my favourite books of poems around and pick them up and visit them again and again.

I have always had my belief in God but I suppose I just took it for granted. At times when life was busy I could go for days without uttering a prayer of any sort. Of course, when I fell ill I immediately began the begging prayers, looking for God to relieve me of my cancer and make everything all right. But as I tried to come to terms with my illness and what my future might bring I felt myself turning more to God for support to deal with what was coming and I built a closer relationship with God that remains to this day.

All these strategies were used in that first year along with many others but I have also carried many of them into my daily life now. Though I feel well in myself once again and have returned to a more normal daily life, I am still made aware of my illness by the necessity of regular visits to the hospital for check ups and the ongoing medication I have to take.

When I run upstairs now I try to remember the time that I used to stand at the bottom of the stairs and look at them as if they were Mount Everest. At those times I often despaired of my ability to ever get to the top. Without dwelling too much on that time, I find that it is good to keep those memories and realise that life can be lived at a slower pace. I try to remember to slow down and appreciate what I have. So now I cut corners when I can on all the unnecessary things. I try to make time for what I consider the important things in my life. This is the only shot I am going to get at it and having been given a reprieve I am determined to enjoy as much of it as I can.

In serious illness you need to make both short-term and long-term changes to your lifestyle to help your well-being.

Learn from your strategies and adopt some of them permanently.

You get one shot at life so it makes sense to prioritise. Not every task has to be done.

Find your own ways to cut corners.

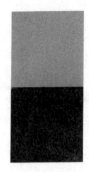

chapter 13

In for the Long Haul: Coping with the Bad Days

Shortly after my surgery, I woke in the middle of the night in pain. My right arm felt swollen and my right side felt as if it was going to burst. I lay in the dark for a while with all sorts of wild imaginings flitting through my head until I thought it would burst also. I got up and went downstairs. Sitting in an armchair at 3.00 a.m. in the morning I felt so alone. I knew that I could call my husband and talk it out with him, that I wasn't really alone, but I also knew that the fear was inside of me and that I would have to find a way to cope with it. I sat there for a while and prayed a little, calling on God to help me handle this. I also tried to reason with myself, telling myself that I wasn't really going to suddenly explode on the spot.

That early morning now seems a long time ago, yet there have been many times since then when a similar panic has returned and I have had to live with this.

There are the days when I get the unexplained pain and up pops the question of whether the cancer is back; the times when my head spins with the question of what I will do if it returns.

Everybody has their bad days. The days when we don't want to get out of the bed or the days that we do get up and wish we hadn't. We all need our coping mechanisms to deal with these. Being seriously ill just adds another dimension to the situation.

I have found that reading books on how other people dealt with these situations is very helpful for me. We cannot but admire people who have faced great adversity and moved through it. It may not necessarily be illness, it can be any life situation that brings us down and makes living difficult. The story of the courage others show and how they get past the limitations their lives impose on them always gives me a lift.

I once read a quote found by Allied soldiers at the end of World War II scratched on a basement wall when they entered a bombed-out building in Germany. It had been left there by victims of the Holocaust:

I believe in the sun – even when
it does not shine
I believe in love – even when it
is not shown
I believe in God – even when he
does not speak.

For me, coping with my bad days is like believing in the sun even when it doesn't shine. It is trying to have faith that when the day or even weeks are bad, there is a sun there somewhere and that it will shine again.

Recently the son of a friend had a sporting accident in which he broke his leg. Trying to find ways to make life okay for a child who is encased in plaster for six weeks is a difficult task. My friend remarked to me that she felt somewhat ashamed of being out of sorts with this situation when others were much worse off and dealing with more long-term situations. But it doesn't really matter what the illness is or how long its duration. If we were to start to compare ourselves to others there is always someone worse off than we are. That means nothing when we are suffering; the illness we have to deal with is the one that concerns us. It is the one that we need to find the coping mechanisms for.

Some days coping means just that. You get up in the morning, and sometimes that is a real act of courage in itself, and you struggle through the day as best you can. I find that on the bad days it helps to try to put in my best effort to show a well-turned-out me to the world. If I can look better on the outside it helps a little with how I am feeling on the inside. Sometimes the window dressing is important.

I also have to remind myself that there is no reason why I should have a clear run through life with nothing to disturb the calm surface of my existence. Instead of asking the question, 'Why me?', the question I try to ask myself now is, 'Why not me?' Many bad things happen to good people and we have to find our way to deal with that.

If you find something that helps you cope or that lifts your spirits, make a note of it and keep it as part of your survival strategies that I talked about in the previous chapter.

There is an excerpt from a poem by William Blake entitled 'Auguries of Innocence' that I find helps me on days when I am really down:

It is right it should be so:
Man was made for Joy and
Woe
And when this we rightly know
Thro' the world we safely go.

MAIN POINTS

Try to have faith that the bad days will pass – that the sun is there even if you can't see or feel it.

Don't feel guilty for being out of sorts. Allow yourself to acknowledge that you are feeling down.

Bad things happen to good people – that's part of life.

---

in for the long haul

chapter 14

Keeping a Sense of Self – I am Still Me

When you are diagnosed with a serious illness a lot of changes take place. I have already talked about some of the things that might happen. Some of the changes can be within you, both physically and emotionally. The changes can also come from without; some people immediately begin to see you differently and can even show this without realising what message they are giving to you.

With all of this going on it can sometimes be very hard to hold on to the core of who you are. We cannot get away from the reality that illness does bring many changes and sometimes there are adjustments to be made, but this doesn't mean that we have to lose our true selves.

When I was ill the immediate and first step that needed to be taken was a mastectomy. I knew that this was necessary to stop the spread of the cancer but knowing that didn't make it any easier to accept. In our modern society bodily appearances can be very important and we feel that we are, to a certain extent, judged by them. Shortly after the operation I had to go for a course of chemotherapy and that led to my hair falling out. In the space of a few months I had gone from being an average-looking woman in her mid-forties to what, I felt, was a freak with one breast and no hair. I felt sure that if people could see me without the protection of prosthesis and wig they would be disgusted by me.

During those months when I wore a wig I dreaded windy days and had bad dreams of the wig suddenly flying off and that I would be left standing bare-headed for all to see. I kept telling myself that these were minor things, and that the fight to save my life was what I should be thinking of. But when I was coping with the possibility of this, it was very difficult to face this loss of self-image as well.

These were my personal horrors but everybody dealing with a serious illness has their own issues to deal with. We all have our stories of how hard it can be to hang on to our essential selves, how we find it hard to convince ourselves and others that we are still the person we were. It is difficult not to see our lives in terms of pre- and post-illness and sometimes we can start to define ourselves in this context.

At a time like this we are made to examine who we really think we are and what it is about ourselves that we value. One thing that I had plenty of was time, as a lot of my normal daily activities had to be put on hold. When you have time on your hands you can be forced to ask questions that you usually try to avoid.

In order to hang on to your sense of self when you are ill you need to know what it is you are hanging on to and also you need to decide the true worth of these things that you value so much. In an earlier chapter I talked about the guilt feeling I had when I fell ill. While feeling guilty is of no value in itself, it is valuable in assessing your lifestyle and seeing how it works for you.

The changes that occur are both physical and emotional, and sometimes we can feel slightly ashamed when we get upset about some physical change that takes place. I felt that I should be glad that I was alive and that I was being given another chance at life. Getting upset about a temporary loss of hair seemed shallow. But shallow or not at that time, having to lose my hair and wear a wig just seemed one more thing to bear.

Seven years on my hair is back but I will always have to deal with what I still regard as a disfigurement to my body, my mastectomy. Yet I have adjusted to life as I am and if it is a choice between losing a breast or losing my life then there is no contest. Of course, given the choice I wish I was back to before the time I found that lump and all the consequences that came from that discovery, but I have discovered strength within myself that I didn't think I possessed.

I have learned that my true self is not defined by my body shape, or by how others perceive me. Somebody seeing me in a certain way does not mean I am that way. I am who I always was and will continue developing because of all my life experiences. My illness was and is part of these experiences but my life is so much more than that.

I turned fifty a couple of years ago and as I celebrated my birthday with family and friends I was truly thankful for all I have in my life. I know that I am a product of all the experiences I have had in my life so far and the experiences to come, both good and bad, will continue to change and mould me. My self-image will continue to change and grow and this is how it should be.

Try to define your sense of self, what it is about yourself that you value.

Do not be ashamed that some things to do with your illness upset you. If anything causes you pain, it is important and relevant.

We constantly change and grow throughout our life and our illness is only part of this changing and growing; we are more than our illness.